Live Right!

Beating Stress in College and Beyond

Debra Atkinson

Iowa State University

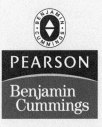

PEARSON

Benjamin
Cummings

San Francisco Boston New York
Cape Town Hong Kong London Madrid Mexico City
Montreal Munich Paris Singapore Sydney Tokyo Toronto

Acquisitions Editor: Sandra Lindelof
Project Editor: Alison Rodal
Development Manager: Claire Alexander
Managing Editor: Deborah Cogan
Production Supervisor: Caroline Ayres
Production Management and Compositor: WestWords, Inc.
Interior Designer: Jeanne Calabrese
Cover Designer: Jeanne Calabrese

Photo Researcher: Clare Maxwell
Director, Image Resource Center: Melinda Patelli
Image Rights and Permissions Manager: Zina Arabia
Manufacturing Buyer: Stacy Jenson
Executive Marketing Manager: Neena Chandra
Text printer: R.R. Donnelley/Harrisonburg
Cover printer: R.R. Donnelley/Harrisonburg

Credits

Cover photo: LWA-Dann Tardif/zefa/Corbis; **41** Bruce Laurence/Getty Images; **57** Colin Hawkins/Getty Images; **58** Altrendo Images/Getty; **60** John Giustina/Getty Images; **63** Erik Dreyer/Getty Images; **71** Blasius Erlinger/Getty Images; **iii, v, 1, 2, 3, 5, 9, 13, 15, 16 17, 18, 19, 21, 23, 24, 28, 30, 31, 32, 33, 35, 39, 40, 44, 45, 46, 47, 48, 49, 51, 52, 53, 59, 61, 62, 64, 65, 66, 67, 68, 69, 72** Getty Images; **8, 10, 13, 29, 70** Corbis; **30, 52, 61** SuperStock

Library of Congress Cataloging-in-Publication Data
Atkinson, Debra.
  Live right! : beating stress in college and beyond / Debra Atkinson. — 1st ed.
    p. cm.
  ISBN 0-321-49149-1 (pbk.)
  1. College student orientation. 2. Stress management. I. Title.
  LB2343.3.A86 2008
  378.19'8—dc22

                        2006031407

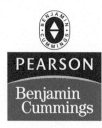

www.aw-bc.com

ISBN 13: 978-03214-9149-7
ISBN 10: 0-321-49149-1
19 20 — DOH—17 16 15

Contents

Preface

Hundreds of students in my Health Studies course had a significant impact on the content of this book. They have educated me in what I can do to help them deal better with their stressors, as they candidly shared personal experiences throughout their semester. Students from a variety of majors all report very similar stressors while in college. Exploring ways to deal with stress and enhance your coping skills is what this book is all about. My hope is that you read this book and can put some of the tools and ideas to use immediately.

Many experts assist me in teaching the Health Studies course by sharing their wisdom in my classroom. Many of them have planted seeds and given me the ideas included here in this book. Generously, they discussed stress-coping techniques with me and helped to turn this into practical steps for dealing with stress. This was most definitely a group project.

Stress doesn't go away. While you have a heartbeat, you will have some stress. Finding ways to reduce or eliminate the *distress* in your life is the goal. I hope that you understand the power that you have over stress and know that by taking action, even in picking up this book and opening to a chapter, you can begin to feel better.

Unfortunately, there aren't guidelines or position statements on stress busting. With exercise or nutrition, you can find guidelines based on your age and gender and your goals. As you work on your stress-busting plan, you'll be finding the right fit for you. You are the expert here. Explore what works for you. Consider information from others, and listen to what works for them, but ultimately you will choose for yourself your own stress-busting blueprint.

The importance of what you learn here goes far beyond how you do on any exam. The real value is on what you take with you for the rest of your life.

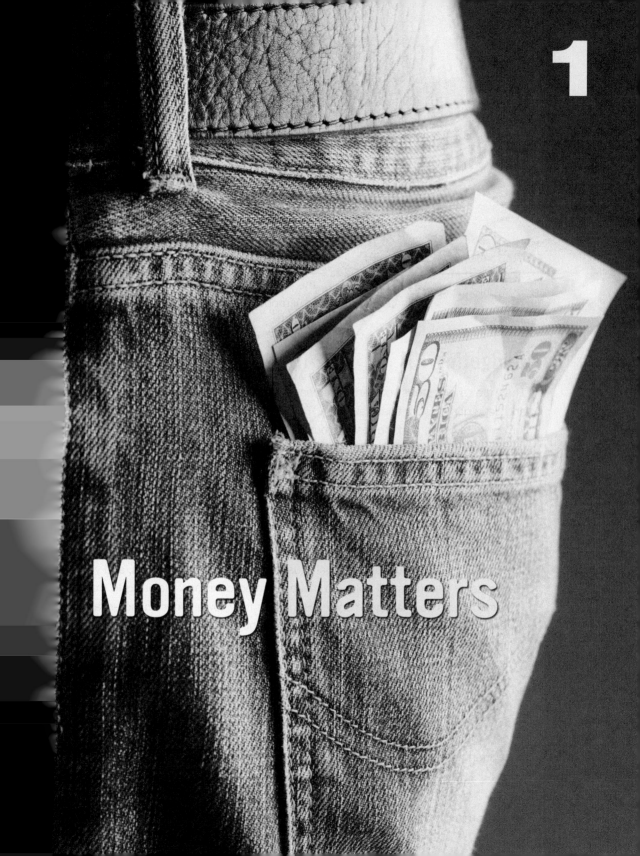

Money Matters

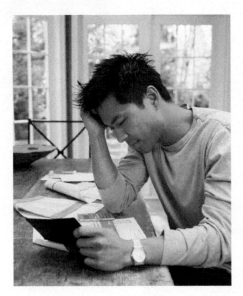

Whether you've been managing your own finances for twenty days or twenty years, money can be a significant source of stress. As a college student, you are probably managing your money all on your own, from checking accounts, to credits cards, to budgeting for a night out, for the first time. You might feel confused, have negative feelings about managing your finances, or just ignore the issue altogether. Careful planning and developing skills to cope with tight times can help you lower your money-related stress level. If you are on your own for the first time, the tips in this chapter will help you manage your money, instead of it managing you!

Budgeting 101

There are several steps you can implement to get a handle on your actual expenses and get a grip on your financial status. These "budget basics" will be useful to you throughout college and the rest of your life. Consider each step described below, then look at the worksheet example on pages 3–5. Create your own worksheet just like this to get a grip on your budget.

1. **Create awareness.** If you avoid keeping track of your financial status because you may find it depressing to learn you have $10.00 in your checking account, you are not alone. Many students who take this approach know they don't have a lot of money and may not see the point in making it go a little further. Being knowledgeable about your financial situation, your spending patterns, and your necessary expenses will help you make informed decisions. Refusing to make hard choices to manage money responsibly may lower your finance-related stress level now, but come the first of every month, you might find yourself in crisis mode. On the other hand, an awareness of what you have in your bank account, what you owe to the credit card company, and how much you need to spend on things like books and food will make you feel more in control now and help you create lifelong habits for successful money management. To become aware of where your money goes on a daily basis, *complete Step 1 of the budget worksheet* by tracking your spending habits for one month. Don't include recurring expenses just yet; we'll get to those in a few more steps.

Sample Budget Worksheet

Wonder why you barely break even at the end of the month? Trying to save for spring break? Use this worksheet as an example of how to track your spending habits and determine a budget. Do this for four weeks to get a true idea of how you spend your money.

Step 1: Where does your money come from?

Here, log all of your sources of income for the month. Include money you earn working, loan checks, gifts, and any other sources of income you have.

INCOME		SOURCE
Week 1	$100.00	Pay day!
Week 2	$1,000.00	Financial aid
Week 3	$100.00	Birthday money
Week 4	$500.00	Mom and Dad
Total	$1,700.00	

Step 2: Where does your money go?

Make a list of your daily, out-of-pocket expenses. What counts? Do include things like going to the movies, dining out, concert tickets, clothing purchases, and trips to Starbucks. Don't include recurring purchases like rent, gas, books, and other things you pay for every week, month, or semester.

AMOUNT SPENT		PURPOSE
Week 1	$10.00	Movie
	$5.00	Lunch at campus
	$50.00	New shoes
	$6.00	Lattes
	$10.00	Dinner out
Week 1 total	$86.00	

continued

Sample Budget Worksheet (continued)

	AMOUNT SPENT	PURPOSE
Week 2	$8.00	Sunday breakfast
	$4.00	Notebook and pens
	$13.00	Lunch in student center
	$45.00	Concert ticket
	$5.00	Sodas from dorm vending machine
	$6.00	Lattes

Week 2 total $81.00

	AMOUNT SPENT	PURPOSE
Week 3	$35.00	New shirt for date on Friday
	$3.00	Postage for notes to grandparents
	$20.00	Snacks for movie night
	$10.50	Movie rentals
	$18.00	Cosmetics

Week 3 total $86.50

Total for month: $253.50

Step 3: Now record your fixed expenses

Record your fixed expenses, or those things you know you have to shell out for every week, month, or semester. Break it down into months if you can, so if you have things you pay for once a semester, divide the total by 4, or if you have things you pay for weekly, multiply the weekly total by 4.

WEEKLY		MONTHLY		SEMESTER	
Gas	$50.00	Rent	$400.00	Tuition	$2,500.00
Groceries	$60.00				
Total	$110.00	Total	$400.00	Total	$2,500.00

Monthly total: $1,465.00

Sample Budget Worksheet (continued)

Step 4: Do the math

Total up your income and then your fixed expenses. Now subtract your monthly fixed expenses from your monthly income.

(Step 1) – (Step 3) = what you have left over for out-of-pocket expenses, or for saving a little extra

$1,700.00	(income)
– $1,465.00	(fixed expenses)
$235.00 =	how much money you have for out-of-pocket spending each month

You're almost there! Now look at what you have left each month above, and compare this amount to Step 2. Is your Step 2 total greater? Are you shocked or surprised at how much you spend without even really thinking about it? How can you use this information to improve your spending habits?

2. **Income.** Believe it or not, you have income even if you don't work. When you assess your income, consider money you receive from financial aid loans, gifts, work, your parents, or other sources. *This is the second step on the budget worksheet,* so again, look at the example on page 3, then start your own log of your monthly income. If you aren't working right now but think you'd like to have extra money to spend, getting a part-time job on campus or somewhere close by might be an option you want to consider. Don't be afraid to get creative. Could you tutor other students in a class you are strong in? Maybe you love pets or children, and could pet-sit or babysit. You could also trade a skill you have. For example, could you do small repairs or main-tenance at your apartment complex in exchange for reduced rent?

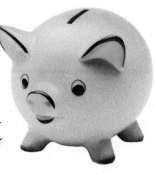

Budget Worksheet

Use this blank worksheet, following the example on pages 3–5, to assess
your finances for one month.

Step 1: Where does your money come from?

Step 2: Where does your money go?

Budget Worksheet (continued)

Step 3: Now record your fixed expenses.

Step 4: Do the math.

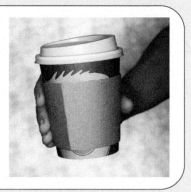

3. Expenses. Have you ever opened your wallet only to discover that the $20.00 bill you were sure you had is gone? Examining where your money goes can be an eye-opening experience. First, everyone has fixed expenses (expenses you cannot avoid) in order to take care of necessities. As a student, fixed expenses occur on both a semester and monthly basis. Each semester brings your tuition bill, book purchases, and course supplies. On a monthly basis you may have rent, utility bills, and car insurance. There will always be the desire to purchase something you don't really need, but you have to make choices. To evaluate how much money you need on a monthly basis to cover your necessities, *follow the example in Step 3 of the budget worksheet.* Track these expenses for a full month. If you have weekly expenses, multiply them by 4. If you have semester expenses, divide those by 4 to get a grip on how much you need to save each month to cover those costs when the time comes.

8

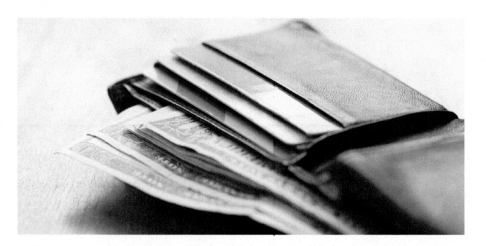

Sticking to your planned budget

Avoiding temptation is key to controlling your spending habits. You've already considered the potential money you can spend on incidentals if you're not careful. Even bigger purchases can mean even bigger problems. Like any behavior change plan, if you do want better control of your money, consider the obstacles along the way. You might want to buy clothes, go on a vacation, or spend money going out with friends; this doesn't go away just because the pocketbook is tight.

What are some specific obstacles you face? Do you walk by your favorite shoe store on your way to class each day? Does your roommate call and ask if you want to go shopping? Do you go online browsing? A small shot of "retail therapy" can cause a big overspending headache when you get your credit card bill or don't have enough money to pay rent.

Table 1.1 Curb Spontaneous Spending

Do you spend your money on . . .	Savings tip
sodas from the dormitory vending machine?	Rather than spend up to $1.50 every day, buy a case of soda at the grocery store and save.
a daily cup of coffee at your favorite coffee shop?	Buy a travel mug and brew your own at home.
candy bars to munch on while studying?	Try buying healthy and more economical snacks, like bags of carrots, apples, or other snack foods in bulk.
magazines?	If you and your friends have similar taste in magazines, consider buying a subscription, which often saves you a lot of money compared to buying one issue, and split the cost.
eating out?	Consider visiting your university's cafeteria more often, or making low-cost creations in the dorm. A meal plan that allows you two visits to the cafeteria each day (breakfast and lunch) could save you some money on dining out and groceries.

Consider giving yourself a rule in order to avoid impulse buying. For example, make it a rule not to buy something you didn't intend to purchase right away. Write down the item you want and the cost. If it is a big-ticket item, give it a week to think it over; if it's a smaller item, give it three days. When the time is up, you will have been able to weigh if you really want to buy it or not.

If you do decide to go, or can't avoid it, go with a purpose, or a specific shopping goal in mind. For example, if you have a genuine need for new shoes, stick to the plan! Don't start trying on pants instead. Here are some other tips for avoiding a shopping spree:

- Determine in advance if and how much you'll spend.

- Imagine saying no to a clerk.

- Use positive affirmations to support your choices, like "I am choosing to spend my money more wisely," or ask yourself, "Do I really want this, or do I want to save for spring break?"

- Use cash or your debit card. It is immediate, and it's gone. One caveat to debit card use: make sure you do not have overdraft protection. It will go into effect if you don't have the funds for a purchase, and it usually carries a hefty fee.

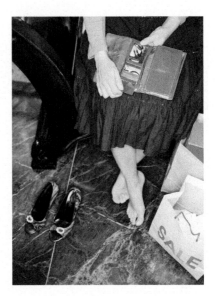

Credit Cards: Show Me the Plastic!

Credit card offers are abundant. They find their way into your mailbox, your book bag, and your bank statement. The convenience of a credit card is one huge advantage of carrying them. They are especially useful if you are away from home, traveling, or making purchases online. They also allow you to establish a credit record for future purchases. The temptation to spend money you don't actually have is an obvious disadvantage. This is a temptation too great for many: college students have an average credit card debt of $5,500.00 at graduation. Is it any wonder plastic can cause such stress? It doesn't have to, but you have to know your spending habits and how to use your credit card responsibly.

Credit card companies like students. If they can get you to use their credit card, they know you might use that card for your entire life. They also consider your parents to be an added guarantee that your bill will get paid. Consider the following when choosing a credit card.

Interest rates

How high is it? Look at the section that says *APR* on the terms and conditions before you apply. At the time of this writing, anything below 10% is good. You'll be charged this percentage of interest on any balance you carry each month, unless you pay in full. Also, is the APR variable or fixed? Fixed APR is a better choice. If the interest rate is varied, read the fine print and highlight it so that you understand what might cause the interest rate to increase. For instance, credit card companies can change fixed interest rates to variable ones, even if they originally promised you the fixed rate. They only have to send you a notification that within a short period your rate will change. As a credit card user you will be given an opt-out form to avoid the rate change, but would still pay the new interest if you carried a balance on the card in the future.

Late payment fees

Make sure you know what this is. Though it is good practice to always pay your bill on time, be aware of what you will be charged if you do pay late. Also know that each late payment will show up on your credit report.

Credit Speak

Annual Fee A fee your credit card company might charge you on a yearly basis.

APR (Annual Percentage Rate) Yearly percentage rate charged when a balance is held on a credit card. Applied each month when an outstanding balance is present.

Balance Transfer Fee Credit card charge for transferring a balance from one account to another. This fee is often a percentage of the balance you want to transfer.

Credit Limit Total amount that can be charged on a card.

Grace Period Time allowed for paying without being charged a late and/or finance fee.

Finance Charge Fees billed to you for a balance transfer, as part of late fees, as over-the-limit fees, or as a portion of what you are charged when you carry a balance from month to month (interest).

Fixed Rate APR Annual Percentage Rate that does not change throughout the year.

Prime Rate (Prime Interest Rate) Rate at which banks lend to most creditworthy customers. Known to change, but not on a regular basis. Variable rate cards change according to this national rate.

11

Annual fees

Some credit cards charge you an annual fee, but usually only if it is a special "rewards" card. It can be as little as $30.00, but could be $75.00 or higher. Make sure you know this information before signing up. There are plenty of credit cards that don't have annual fees, so don't feel that you must choose one that does.

Identity theft and insurance

This is something to consider. Does your credit card have this option? How do you make a claim if your card is lost or stolen? Choose cards that offer this protection automatically without requiring you to pay a fee for this type of protection.

Want to learn more? At www.creditcards.com you can search, compare, and apply for credit cards online. Once you've identified a few credit cards that look good to you, use the worksheet below to compare each one, looking at all of the points mentioned above.

Credit Card Comparison

Use this worksheet to compare card offers side by side. Some features may not be as important to you as others. If you are disciplined and pay off your card each month, interest rate matters less. If you are getting out of debt, 0% APR introductory rates and low fixed interest rates are important.

	INTEREST RATE	IS THE INTEREST RATE VARIABLE OR FIXED?	LATE PAY PENALTY	ANNUAL FEE
Card 1				
Card 2				
Card 3				
Card 4				
Card 5				

Credit Card Q & A

What is credit history, and why is it important?

Generally, the best rule of thumb in using credit cards is to pay off the balance in full and on time each month. Some people might want to establish credit history, though, which basically would show a bank or other lender that you are a good risk when the time comes for you to purchase a home or a car. Credit cards are a way to establish the proof that you can have a bill and pay consistently over time. Experts recommend leaving a small balance on your account by not paying it off in full for several months in a row to establish good credit history.

How is my credit limit determined?

Remember that credit card companies make their money when you pay interest. When you are a new customer, your credit limit might be very low. Over time, they may "reward" you for doing business with them by increasing your credit limit. To avoid racking up debt, ask instead for a small credit limit. You are the only one really taking care of your money. If something sounds too good to be true, be sure to ask yourself if it is a good idea.

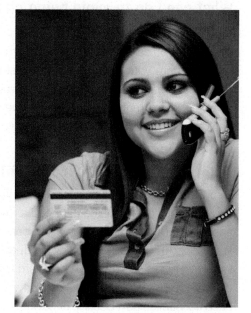

Are those department store credit cards a good idea?

The cashier rings up your new jeans and asks if you want to save 10% on your purchase today by applying for a credit card. Should you or shouldn't you? Experts agree that store credit cards usually aren't the best. They have even higher APRs than major credit cards do, making it wise to pay off that balance right away. The promised special coupons and offers never come, but they know that your likelihood of spending more does.

The bigger disadvantage is that too many credit cards will have a negative effect on that credit history you are trying to build, and could impact your loan for a car or home should you need one. If you are making a big purchase and want to take advantage of the 10% discount, the best thing to do is pay the bill when it arrives and then cancel the card immediately.

What is the maximum number of credit cards I should have?

Two major credit cards are reasonable. You should use only one, but it may be wise to have the second on hand for emergencies. Occasionally, your credit card company may track your spending habits, and if you are using a card in a way that is not consistent with your normal usage (for example, using it daily because you are traveling), the company might close the card temporarily as part of their fraud protection action. You don't want to be on spring break planning to use your one credit card, and suddenly not have that as an option.

What can I do to avoid being charged late payment fees?

Avoid late payment fees and increasing interest rates by making automatic online payments. You can set up your credit card account online, and set up an automatic payment from your checking account straight to your credit card for a specific amount and date. If you have any concerns about the safety of paying online, consider that many more people shop online with their credit card number, and your bank's online service is certainly more safe than that.

What are my alternatives to carrying a credit card?

Debit cards are widely used today and with big advantages. This plastic form of your own money eliminates the need for writing checks and carrying cash, yet still ensures that the money is there to spend, unlike credit cards. You can even use your debit/ATM card like a credit card, as most carry either a Visa or MasterCard logo. Make sure you still have a system for recording your purchases to track your current balance. Determine what works best for you, whether it be writing down each transaction as it occurs, or saving receipts and tallying them up once a week.

2

Finding the Time
Balancing College Life

When was the last time you pulled an all-nighter because it was the only time you could find to study for your exam the next day? Have you ever felt like you have so much to do that you don't even know where to begin? Do you have trouble fitting homework, a social life, and your part-time job into a regular day?

You might find college life challenging because it is so unstructured. You enjoy the freedom of college and yet find that planning time to study, work, socialize, and exercise is all up to you for the first time. Gone are the study halls, parents to monitor your work schedule and ask you if you've done your homework, and planned social and sports activities. Now that you are living on your own, it's up to you to decide what you *need* to do now, what you *want* to do now, and what can wait until later.

What does *time management* mean? It's a term you probably hear a lot these days from professors, academic advisors, and older students who aren't new to the college game. You literally have 24 hours in a day and 168 hours in a week, including time for sleep, and how you choose to spend this time is up to you. It comes down to knowing what your priorities are. This chapter will help you assess all of the things you may need to do each day, and help you prioritize between schoolwork, friends, and your job, while still making sure you've got some time for yourself, sleep, and meals. You can't add hours to the day, but you can learn how to get the most of the time you've got.

Deciding What to Do and When to Do It

Determining what is important to you is an important first step in managing your time wisely. Although your priorities might change slightly on a daily basis, you are probably spending the most time on things that mean the most to you. Sometimes what is most important isn't always clean, cut, and dry. What do you do when getting an A on your biology exam tomorrow is a goal you have, but your new friends are going to the football game and bonding with them is also important to you? It isn't always easy to keep your long-term goals in clear sight when you've got to decide how to spend your time. Assessing how important all of your "time takers" are can help you determine what to skip, and what you can't go without doing.

Assess your "time takers"

The worksheet on pages 17–18 will help you take the first step in making the most of the time you have each day. Once you've completed the worksheet, you might find that you aren't using your time that well. The tips in this chapter will help you make the time for the things that matter to you most.

Priority Checklist

Part I

Identify your highest and lowest priorities, using the worksheet below. Rate each of the following on a scale of 1-10, 10 being most important. A 10 would be something that you want to make time for on a daily basis. You would be willing to drop something else in order to make time for a 10. A 1 occurs on an occasional basis without a sense of urgency. Use any number more than once.

- Attending classes or labs _____

- Studying for exams and completing homework assignments _____

- Going to a party with your friends _____

- Attending a family celebration back home, or just visiting with your family _____

- Getting in a regular workout _____

- Working to pay bills or have spending money _____

- Interning or volunteering to enhance your résumé _____

- Church, meditation, or prayer _____

- Time with a significant other _____

continued

Priority Checklist (continued)

- Attending a club or organization meeting _____

- Keeping up with cleaning/laundry _____

- Shopping or running errands _____

- Time out for a manicure or haircut _____

- A long soak in a bath _____

- Marathon television/playing video games _____

- Enjoying a nice meal _____

- Getting enough sleep _____

- Other _____

Part 2

Now, go back through your list and write down how much time you spend in each area during your week. Do you find that your 10's (above) are getting the most time right now? If so, you're on the right track. If what you say is important to you and the ways you spend real time are consistent, you are likely to be living a life consistent with your values, that is, the things that are guiding your long-term life goals.

Recognize the signs of poor time management

1. You put sleep at the bottom of your list and struggle to stay awake in class. Watching for signs and symptoms of poor time management might prompt you to revisit your priorities. For instance, you might rank sleep low on your list of priorities, and rank getting an A in organic chemistry high, but if you can't stay awake in class, you need to adjust your schedule before your lack of sleep earns you a D instead of an A.

2. You lost three pounds during finals week. If you find that you are so busy that you forget to eat, take steps now to make some time for meals. You don't have to spend a lot of time on preparation: eat prepared foods like pre-sliced fruits and vegetables, microwavable soups, or healthy frozen entrées. Or frequent your cafeteria. It doesn't take much time to run in, make a sandwich, and eat it while you study or walk to class. Mealtime might not be a top priority, but good nutrition is a key to getting all the other things done.

3. Your significant other or family feels neglected. If your relationships are suffering because of time constraints, look for ways to make the people you love feel important to you. Balancing commitments; time with friends, family, and partners; and time for yourself is important to your overall health, and this balance is different for everyone. You may need more or less time with friends or alone; it's a matter of finding what works for you.

Let Your Loved Ones Know You Care

- Send a quick e-mail daily to stay in touch until a larger block of time is available.
- Plan a special event with your loved one like a nice dinner, bowling, or something else you both enjoy and can look forward to.
- Talk with your friends, family, and boyfriend or girlfriend, and let them know they are important to you even though you can't spend as much time with them as you'd like.

19

Make Time for You

Spending too much time on the less important things isn't the only source of time-related stress. You might have several important tasks to accomplish and deal with all at once, or you are the type of person who feels compelled to fill up every second of the day with an activity, work, or chore.

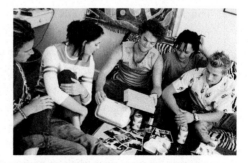

Managing your time wisely includes balancing time with friends with your schoolwork.

When this happens, you can quickly feel overwhelmed, and stress skyrockets. Creating "me time" is an important strategy for coping with stress. The following tips can help you understand the importance of unplanned time and making sure you have some time to yourself.

Strategies to Cope with Time-Related Stress

Coping strategies

1. **Create a schedule.** Use a planner, Palm Pilot, calendar, or any other type of scheduling tool that works for you, and begin by adding only the things that are your greatest priorities and the "fixed time takers." This includes your class schedule, practice or meetings for sports teams or clubs you belong to, commuting time, and study time. If work is a part of your routine, add those hours. Sleep and meals are important, so include these too.

2. **Reserve time for yourself.** Every day, budget an hour of time, beyond resting, that is just for you. This time is meant to recharge your batteries, and should not be spent doing anything you should do or have to do. Do something you enjoy and find relaxing, whether you are alone or with others. If you choose alone time, read a book, go for a walk, or take a nap. With others you might play basketball, get a cup of coffee, or attend a party.

3. **Avoid interruptions.** Roommates will come in and out, and e-mail announcements will flash on the screen. If these distractions will take you off task, plan ahead. For instance, find a spot in the library where you know no one can find

Leave Some "White Space"

"When your life is full, you are missing your life."

Imagine you are in an art gallery the size of a small classroom. How many works of art might you expect to see there? Would the entire wall be covered with art, with no space in between, or would paintings be spread out on a wall? If there is no wall showing between each piece of art, the room will feel crammed and you'll have a difficult time devoting much attention to any single painting. Can you draw some parallels between this visual image, and your life when you try to fill up every single second of your day? The space between the art is as important as the art itself. Without the "white space," viewers fail to appreciate each unique piece. Think of the activities and responsibilities in your life as artwork. Where is your white space? When you prioritize your time and responsibilities, make sure to leave time for you.

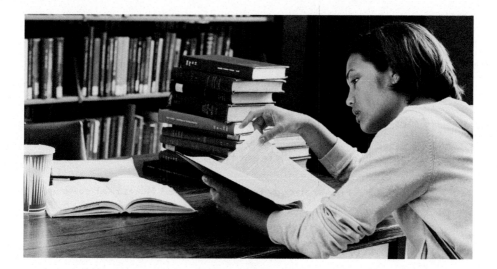

you. Turn off your phone, or the sound on your computer that lets you know you've got new mail. Look back at the schedule you created and be sure you're using dedicated time wisely. If exercise is important to you, set a regular appointment with yourself to get it done.

4. **Pad your time.** Leave yourself a little extra time for error, whether you are trying to complete a paper or meeting someone at a restaurant you've never been to before. Anticipate that things might not always take the exact amount of time you think because you could get lost, or the printer could break moments before your paper is due. Other ways to pad your time include the following: if an assignment is due on Friday, intend to have it done by Wednesday; on a daily basis, try to arrive 10 minutes early to class or to work. Rushing can cause stress—so avoid getting yourself into these types of situations.

5. **Create systems.** For tasks that you do repeatedly, have a system in place that allows you to save time. Instead of running to the store for a birthday card at the last minute, for instance, set aside some time every month or two to buy a set of birthday, anniversary, or blank cards that can work for any occasion. Stock up on postage. When you do your regular supply shopping, buy doubles of items you use all the time like toothpaste, shampoo, and soap or laundry detergent. If you prepare meals for yourself, take an hour once a week to do as much advance preparation as you can, like cutting up vegetables, or making and freezing items that can easily be warmed up in the microwave. If you scramble at the last minute getting out the door in the morning, establish a habit of taking 15 minutes before bed to get your school items, keys, and other essentials ready for the next day.

Time Management Self-Test

Answer yes or no to the following questions.

Yes No

1. ☐ ☐ I tend to rush to get things done at the last minute.

2. ☐ ☐ I react strongly to the unexpected things that come up.

3. ☐ ☐ I find myself getting very upset or irritated when people let me down, miss deadlines, or do less than optimal work.

4. ☐ ☐ I usually arrive rushed or in a hurry.

5. ☐ ☐ I drive over the speed limit, tailgate, or criticize other drivers.

6. ☐ ☐ I tend to arrive late, even if it's not my fault.

7. ☐ ☐ It is difficult to focus on any one thing at a time for very long.

8. ☐ ☐ While I am in class, I am often making lists of what else I need to do.

9. ☐ ☐ I often say "yes" to things I don't really have time to do.

10. ☐ ☐ I almost never have free time just for me.

11. ☐ ☐ It's hard to enjoy relationships because I am constantly thinking about how much I have to do.

If you answered yes to five or more of these, you could benefit from the time management strategies in this chapter.

6. **Learn to say no.** Saying "yes" when you mean to say "no" costs you a lot, and can be a huge source of stress. Practice saying "no." If you find yourself reluctant, defer with "Let me think about it and check my schedule." You'll have time to consider what's best for you without the pressure of the moment. If you are already time-starved, you may want to shelve the following until you have more time:

- Leadership positions in organizations
- Volunteer positions that don't directly benefit you or your career
- Professional organizations that won't help your career
- Social events and activities you only feel obligated to attend
- Romantic goals or pressure you have or someone else is putting on you

7. **Choose multitasking wisely.** In theory, multitasking gets a lot of things done at once. In reality, nothing gets done as efficiently or effectively. A good rule of thumb when choosing to multitask is to try and combine two tasks that don't require too much of your attention. For example, if you want to catch a movie while you are folding towels and matching socks, nothing is going to suffer. On the other hand, you might not want to combine a high-value task like studying for a midterm with watching a movie.

8. **Be in the present moment.** In other words, stay tuned! While you are in class, if you drift off thinking of lunch or you're thirsty or have to go to the bathroom, you are not really there. If you are making a list of things you have to do next, you are not going to get what information you need from the lecture, and it will result in more time outside of class. When you find you are thinking about something other than what you are doing at the moment, remind yourself to tune back in by running to get a drink of water, or simply take notes more actively to stay engaged.

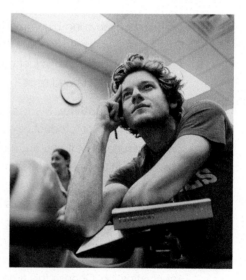

9. **Cut the clutter.** Many of us hang onto stacks of mail, including bills and catalogs, old newspapers, notebooks from last semester, or other items because we want to look at them later, or worry we might need them in the future. Decide immediately if it is worth keeping or not. Do you really need that latest catalog? When was the last time you referenced last semester's biology notebook? If it's worth keeping, act on it now, or file it away in a safe place. If it isn't, throw it in

Table 2.1 Take Back Your Time Checklist

Incorporate the tips into your daily life to make time-management less stressful.

- Leave early, arrive early, and return early. Strive for 10 minutes each.

- Have at least one free hour every day.

- Say "no" to things that don't match directly with your priorities and values.

- Only promise what you know you can deliver easily. Underpromise to overdeliver.

- Plan ahead and be efficient.

- Acknowledge that time is a gift. You choose who to give it to.

- Create systems for tasks you do regularly.

- Leave extra time daily for hassles and emergencies.

24

the trash or recycling bin immediately. Get rid of the "maybe later" or "just in case" pile. If you tend to save things, ask yourself when was the last time you used a certain item that is just collecting dust. Chances are, if it has been a few months, you don't need it.

10. **Plan for productivity.** Many of us are naturally most productive at a certain time of day. If you are more productive in the morning, use it to your advantage and plan to do activities, homework, or chores at this time. Likewise, if you prefer to burn the midnight oil, use this time in a productive manner and avoid procrastination. Choose this time to complete tasks that you might not enjoy, since you know you'll be more motivated, and thus less likely to put them off until the last minute.

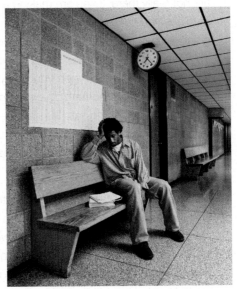

11. Set time limits and balance your day. We are all faced with tasks that we don't enjoy, as well as those that we do enjoy. Balance your day between the two and break up the time you spend on each. If you hate cleaning the bathroom, or paying your bills, tell yourself you'll spend one hour on the less desirable task, followed by one hour of watching your favorite television show. Not only will this help you power through the unpleasant task and avoid monotony, but you'll have a nice reward at the end.

Create Your Core Schedule

Any successful time management plan relies on scheduling. You might think back on your last week and feel unsure about where to begin. The best place to start is with your core activities, or those that you know are fixed and will occur at the same time on a given day of the week. Creating a weekly planner each semester will help you map out your weeks and make the most of each day. This way, when an unexpected curveball comes your way, you'll quickly know how you can fit it in. If your core activities change (for example, you drop a class or join a sports team that meets regularly), create a new schedule. Here are a few additional tips for filling in your weekly planner:

- List all of the courses you are taking on a sheet of paper.
- List extracurricular activities such as clubs, study sessions, work, or sports.
- Schedule time for sleep and meals.
- Leave some free time open (usually the weekend) for recreation and "unplanned" time.
- Schedule in some study time. You don't have to decide in advance what course you will use this time for, but you should plan for some study time each day.

Use the example core schedule on page 26 as a guide to completing the blank schedule on page 27. Insert this schedule into your planning tool of choice (palm pilot, planner, calendar) and you'll be on your way to navigating the time demands of college stress free.

Weekly Planner: Sample Core Schedule

	MON	TUE	WED	THU	FRI	SAT	SUN
7–8	7:45 Wakeup/ breakfast	7:00 Wakeup/ breakfast	7:45 Wakeup/ breakfast	7:00 Wakeup/ breakfast	7:30 Wakeup/ breakfast	Sleep in!	
8–9		Swim practice		Swim practice			
9–10	French	Business	French	Business	French		Wakeup/ breakfast
10–11			1-hour Language lab		Homework		Work (4 hours)
11–12	—11:20— Chem. lecture		—11:20— Chem. lecture				
12–1	—12:30— Lunch	Lunch	—12:30— Lunch	Lunch			
1–2	Homework	Health		Health			
2–3							
3–4	Work (4 hours)		Work (4 hours)	—3:20— Chem. lab (2 hours)			Business 101 study group
4–5		Business 101 study group					
5–6							Dinner
6–7		Dinner		Dinner			
7–8	Dinner	Homework	Dinner	Homework			
8–9			Homework				
9–10							
10–11			Study break				
11–12	Bedtime						

Weekly Planner: Sample Core Schedule

	MON	TUE	WED	THU	FRI	SAT	SUN
7–8							
8–9							
9–10							
10–11							
11–12							
12–1							
1–2							
2–3							
3–4							
4–5							
5–6							
6–7							
7–8							
8–9							
9–10							
10–11							
11–12							

27

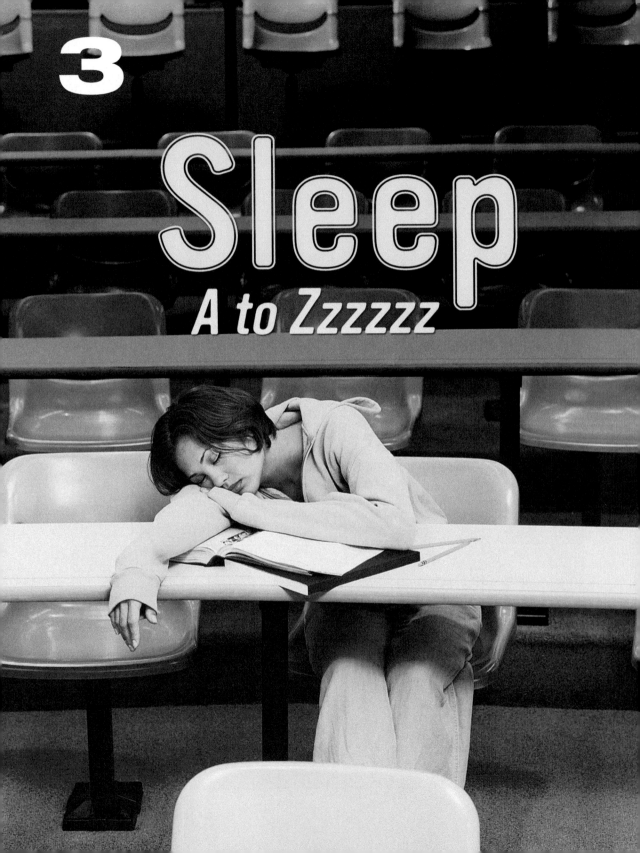

3

Sleep
A to Zzzzzz

It's simple, safe, and free, and getting enough of it is a surefire way to reduce stress levels and put even the biggest crisis into perspective. What is this wonder drug, you ask? Sleep. Want some? Just go to bed a little bit earlier tonight. Quality sleep enhances your ability to cope with stress and is an absolute necessity for optimal health. Easier said than done? Increase your odds of getting the rejuvenating sleep you need by practicing good "sleep hygiene," starting tonight.

Why Is Sleep So Important?

Ever struggled to get some shut-eye while your neighbors partied just outside your dorm room? Have you ever been exhausted yet unable to sleep because you have too many thoughts racing through your head? Lack of sleep can be both a source (like when you can't fall asleep) and a symptom (such as when you've got too much going on in your life) of stress. Sleep deprivation can be a real challenge during college. You might do the following:

- Cheat yourself out of sleep when you can't find enough hours in your day.
- Prioritize studying, sports, and socializing over getting the shut-eye you need.
- Pull the occasional all-nighter since it doesn't seem like one night here and there is that bad.
- Rely on caffeine to help you make it through the day when you are overtired.

What you might not realize is that not only can lack of sleep create undue stress, but also, when you consistently don't get a full night's rest, you become more vulnerable to a wide variety of serious illnesses. It depresses the immune system, making you more likely to catch your best friend's cold or a whole range of other illnesses from strep throat to mononucleosis. Inadequate sleep affects learning, memory, and attention span, all critical to your academic performance. Sure you still want to stay up studying the night before a big exam?

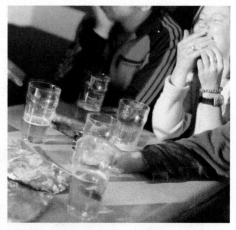

Between classes, homework, and play, it isn't always easy to get the shut-eye you need.

How much sleep do I need?

The amount of sleep we need varies from person to person, but on average a solid 6–8 hours of sleep each night is usually

Sleep Sabotagers

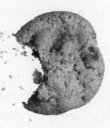

- Partying late into the night, especially if alcohol is used.
- Too much caffeine. Turning to sodas and coffee to offset a bad night's sleep can make the problem even worse the next night.
- Vigorous exercise too close to bedtime.
- Depression, anxiety, or some chronic conditions, and the medications used to treat them.
- Late night snacking. While you don't want to go to bed hungry, a full stomach can keep you up.
- Odd work hours that interfere with your natural body clock, such as working the graveyard shift.

30

enough to allow your body the time it needs to repair itself from the previous day's challenges. Most people don't get enough, though, and usually are anywhere from 30 minutes to 2 hours lacking in the sleep department. College life doesn't help much either. Dorms can be noisy, and you might have papers and projects to complete, or a part-time job to squeeze in on top of it all.

Can I catch up on sleep?

You can, but it isn't easy, and your body knows when you are behind on sleep. When you don't get the optimal amount of sleep your body needs to function at its best, you go into sleep debt, and this debt accumulates over time. Let's say you know you need 8 hours of sleep each night to be at your best, but 5 days a week, you can't seem to get to bed before midnight, and the alarm clock rings at 7:00 A.M. On Friday night, you go to a party with friends and don't make it to bed until 3:00 A.M. On Saturday morning, you've got to be at work by 9:00, so that alarm clock rings at 8:00. By now you have a sleep debt of 8 hours.

Saturday night rolls around, and you go to bed early and wake up on Sunday at your leisure, getting a full 8 hours of sleep. Have you erased your debt? Not so, say the experts. You still need to "catch up" on the 8 hours you lost by getting as much extra sleep as possible. Without catching up, you'll find it hard to feel wide awake or perform at your peak during the day.

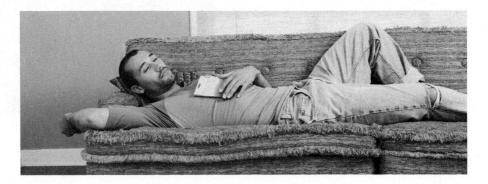

Do you sacrifice sleep to squeeze in all your other daily responsibilities? Want to get out of debt? Try using the National Sleep Foundation's "Sleepiness Diary," found at www.sleepfoundation.org, or use the diary guidelines at the end of this chapter to determine your sleep needs and track your progress toward being debt-free.

Sleep Lessons Learned from a Night Shift Worker

There are many lessons to be learned from those who work nights about good sleep hygiene and why sleep plays an important part in feeling your best. While students might not work the graveyard shift, staying up all night on a regular basis isn't much different.

Changing your body's natural clock

Like people who travel to different time zones, graveyard shift workers must employ a variety of strategies to fool their body into thinking it is daytime when it is dark out and nighttime when the sun rises. If you absolutely have to pull an all-nighter, you can use these tips to help you feel your best. Everyone's body and natural rhythm are different, but you can apply these tips to keep a lack of sleep from stressing you out.

31

1. Extend your sleep time.

If you are able to anticipate a late night ahead of you, try to get to bed extra early the night before, or sleep later than usual if your schedule allows. People who work nights might sleep in late on the day of their night shift to help them cope with the schedule. Try napping too. This extra sleep helps limit your sleep debt.

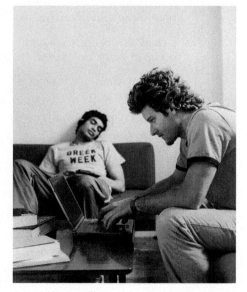

2. Develop a healthy way to make it through the lows.

Graveyard shift workers have what they call the *bewitching hour*, a time of night when you seem to get very tired and need to revive yourself. If you must stay awake, you can try taking a brisk walk or having a healthy snack. Protein can enhance your alertness, and so you can try a glass of milk, a piece of cheese, or some peanut butter on celery or an apple for an energy-packed late night snack. There are also certain foods that will help you sleep. Generally, foods that are high in carbohydrates and calcium and low in protein make the best bedtime snacks. Look at Table 3.1 for the best snooze-inducing snacks.

3. Signal your body to let it know what time of day it is.
Following a night shift, workers head home to get some sleep. It isn't easy, though; even though you've been awake all night, your brain knows that it is light out and it is time to be awake. You have to commit to making sleep a priority and giving cues to your body that will reset its clock. If you pulled an all-nighter or are trying to adjust to a different time zone, try these tips from night workers: If it's light out, wear sunglasses to trick your body into thinking it is dark out, darken the room with blinds, and limit sleep to 2–3 hours so you can get back on a normal day schedule and fall asleep the next night. When it is time to get up, exercise or perform any other activity that signals your body that it is "morning."

Table 3.1 Snacking for Better Sleep

Foods that help you sleep	Foods that keep you awake
• an oatmeal raisin or peanut butter cookie and a glass of milk	• caffeinated foods, including chocolate, hot chocolate, tea, colas, and coffee
• a small slice of apple pie and scoop of vanilla ice cream	• high-fat foods such as a cheeseburger with French fries, or pizza with meat toppings
• a bowl of whole-grain cereal with milk or soymilk	• spicy foods, especially Thai, Indian, and Mexican dishes
• a peanut butter sandwich made with whole-wheat bread	• cured meats such as sausage or pepperoni, and cheeses
• hummus and whole-wheat pita bread	• eggs
• a few slices of turkey on a piece of whole-wheat bread	• candy, junk food, and other high-sugar, processed snack foods
• pasta with parmesan cheese	
• herbal teas such as chamomile	

Table 3.2 The Stages of Sleep

If you are . . .	Then you're in . . .
exhausted no matter how hard you try to stay awake	Stage 1 sleep. Sleep can overtake you. You are not aware you are sleeping; your eyes can even be open. Basically, you are "out of it."
easing into a deeper sleep	Stages 2 and 3 sleep. During progressively deeper sleep, melatonin is released. Melatonin is a naturally occurring hormone that resets the body clock to synchronize metabolic functions with activity and rest.
in a very deep sleep	Stage 4 sleep. This is "Delta sleep." In this stage, human growth hormone (HGH) is released and signals the body to repair worn tissues. Lack of sleep is especially harmful to those who are strength and endurance training, since HGH restores muscles after workouts.
dreaming	Stage 5 sleep. Rapid eye movement (REM) is the stage where you dream. If you lack REM, you become forgetful and irritable. Over-the-counter sleep aids decrease REM, leaving you feeling dazed instead of restored.

33

Why is it important to follow any of this advice?

You, like most college students, probably experience repeated changes in sleep habits and suffer from what feels like chronic "jet lag." It's like having the hangover without the party. Why does this happen? Lack of restorative sleep. Daytime sleep is usually shorter and more often disrupted.

Top Ten Tips for Getting Your Zzzzs

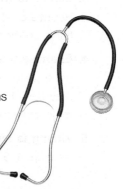

1. **Doctor, doctor.** Rule out the possibility of any health conditions that could contribute to insomnia. Steroids, decongestants, and medications for asthma or depression could have side effects that you want to take into consideration.

Beat Jet Lag

Insomnia, fatigue, stomach ache, or headache; these are symptoms of jet lag and not a great way to spend a spring break vacation. In general, the more time zones you cross, the worse the jet lag. There are ways to avoid or reduce jet lag. Here's how:

- Begin the trip rested (preexisting sleep deprivation intensifies jet lag).
- Plan a daytime flight.
- Reset your watch as soon as you depart.
- Avoid alcohol, caffeine, and nicotine.
- Eat small meals at the appropriate mealtime for your destination.
- Several days before going west: go to bed and wake up 1 hour later each day.
- Once in the west: seek morning light and avoid afternoon light.
- Several days before going east: go to bed and wake up 1 hour earlier each day.
- Once in the east: seek evening light and avoid morning light.
- If you take an overnight flight, avoid sleeping too much on the day of your arrival. You'll find it hard to fight the fatigue, but it will also be harder to adjust to your new time zone's schedule.

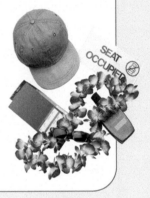

34

2. **Beg, borrow, or steal?** Carefully weigh the advantages of "borrowed" sleep. Many sleep aids, whether prescription or over the counter, interfere with daytime functioning. Safety can be an issue if you are operating a vehicle or even working out with weights in the gym. There also may be a "payback" later when your sleep challenges come back worse than they are now once you stop taking the sleep aid.

3. **Eliminate the villains.** Caffeine, alcohol, and cigarettes all rob you of sleep. Reduce or eliminate them altogether for better sleep. If you also take medications, consider the interaction of these with your meds.

4. **Exercise first, sleep later.** Resist the temptation to put off exercise until you get a good night's sleep. Start slow, but start now. Prepare for days when you may have to reduce your activity level, but keep in mind that regular exercise may help you maintain regular sleep habits.

5. **Timing is everything.** Perform vigorous activity in the late afternoon or early evening, 4–5 hours before bed. Ideally, establish a regular schedule of exercise,

work, and sleep to allow your body to get on a schedule. Also, time meals and snacks so that you are neither hungry nor too full when it's time to hit the hay.

6. **Let there be light.** Spend time in sunlight during the day, especially the mornings when you feel groggy or afternoons when you feel drowsy. Exposure to natural light will have the most positive effects, but turning on the lights and opening the shades will also increase your alertness. You'll be less tempted to nap for too long, which makes getting to sleep at night difficult. Light will delay the production of melatonin, a hormone associated with sleep onset. Melatonin levels that appropriately rise with darkness promote sleep and regular sleep cycles.

7. **All you have to do today is breathe in and breathe out.** Do it deeply. Inhale through your nose to fill your lungs completely, and exhale slowly but completely through slightly pursed lips. Giving your body the oxygen it needs, this breathing technique can also decrease anxiety and tension that make it sometimes difficult to fall asleep. Try five to ten of these deep breaths when your head first hits the pillow.

8. **Tub therapy.** Bathing, like exercise, raises the body temperature. The benefit of doing so is that the decrease in temperature that follows enhances more sound sleep. This imposed thermostat change may help trick your body into sleep. Start running the water 1–2 hours before bedtime. Showers are not quite as effective, but would be better than nothing.

9. **Same time, same place.** Condition yourself into better sleep. Go to bed and rise at the same time. Establish a routine of bedtime rituals that set the stage for sweet dreams. Shower, read, listen to relaxing music, or have a light snack. If thoughts or worries keep you awake, write down anything that you might have on your mind in a "worry journal." Tell yourself, once you've written it down, that you have done all you can until tomorrow. Experiment with what works for you.

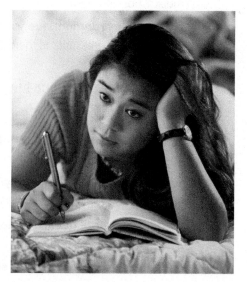

10. **Optimize your sleep environment.** Make the room dark, and not too warm or too cold. If you can't control the noise factor, consider using the "white noise" of a fan to block out disruptive noises.

Weekly Sleep Diary

If you have trouble sleeping, tracking your habits can be a helpful step in identifying factors that might be preventing you from getting your Zzzz's. Use the following guidelines to create your personal sleep diary. A calendar-style diary is shown on the following page.

Part 1: daytime activities and pre-sleep routine

Record the following each night before going to bed.

1. **Food and Drink.** Record only dinner and evening snacks. What did you eat? At what time?

2. **Naps.** Did you nap today? How long did you sleep? Record when and where you napped.

3. **Exercise.** What did you do for exercise today? When? For how long? If you didn't exercise at all, then indicate that.

4. **Medications.** (Include sleep aids.) What types of medications did you take? When did you take them? How often? In what amount?

5. **Alcohol and Caffeine.** Did you drink any alcohol or consume anything containing caffeine? When? How much?

6. **Feelings.** Record how you are feeling emotionally and mentally. Are you happy, sad, anxious, depressed, or stressed? Why?

7. **Bedtime Routine.** What did you do before bed? Relax? Read? Listen to music? For how long?

8. **Bedtime Environment.** Are your bed and pillows comfortable? Is your room too hot/cold, light/dark? Is there noise?

Part 2: Evaluating your sleep

Fill in the details each morning.

1. **How long did it take you to fall asleep?** How did you spend this time? Did you stay in bed and stare at the ceiling? Did you read? Meditate?

2. **Where there interruptions to your sleep?** Did you wake up during the night? If so, what did you do? For how long?

3. **Rate your overall quality of sleep.** Do you feel rested or tired? Was it a good sleep or restless?

4. **Total number of hours spent sleeping** (don't count daytime naps).

Sample Weekly Sleep Diary
Part 1: Daytime Activities and Pre-Sleep Routine

	MON	TUE	WED	THU	FRI	SAT	SUN
Food/Drink							
Naps							
Exercise							
Medications							
Alcohol/ Caffeine							
Feelings							
Bedtime Routine							
Environment							

Part 2: Evaluating Your Sleep

	MON	TUE	WED	THU	FRI	SAT	SUN
How long to fall asleep?							
Interruptions?							
Overall quality of sleep?							
Total sleep hours?							

Making the Grade
Coping with the Demands of School

The cumulative effect of years of looking forward to college, the financial commitment to your education, along with your own and your family's hopes and dreams for your success in college can add up to grade A stress! Like many students, you probably feel like now that you are here, you have to deliver. It isn't always easy, though: you're faced with the unexpected challenges of balancing schoolwork and the demands of your professors with making new friends, adjusting to life away from home, and all the other demands of life that seem to pull you in different direc-

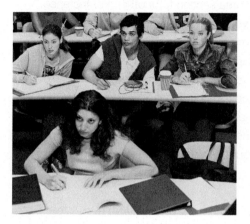

tions. Grades that came easy to you during high school may require more time outside of class than you had expected. Group projects and teamwork are growing parts of course work, and relying on others to do well can create an additional source of academic stress in your life. How will you handle the ups and downs of college life, and the stress your schoolwork may cause? This chapter will give you some solid tips for coping with high expectations, a poor grade, and everything in between.

Be Realistic

Set goals for yourself based on realistic expectations for your exams, courses, and semester grade points. You'll be more satisfied and experience less stress. Sounds simple enough, right? While that seems like a no-brainer, consider the following to establish those realistic expectations.

1. Gather information about your instructors from advisors and other students.
Does a particular professor lecture and use supplemental material in a style that meets your needs? Is the professor available if you need extra help, or does he or she keep regular office hours? Even if the course isn't taught in such a way that works best for you, it will reduce your anxiety to know that your instructor is approachable and willing to help you do your best.

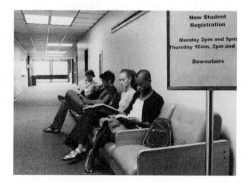

What's Your Learning Style?

Auditory Learners: Learn Best by Listening
If you learn best this way: use a tape recorder in lectures, read text and recite information out loud, and use musical jingles and mnemonic devices to help you remember information.

Visual Learners: Learn Best by Seeing
If you learn best this way: use multiple highlighters or develop other methods to "color code" your notes, take detailed notes, and illustrate ideas to help you understand a concept. Don't be afraid to draw diagrams, charts, maps, graphs, and pictures to help you visualize information.

Tactile/Kinesthetic Learners: Learn Best by Doing
If you learn best this way: chew gum while studying, skim material before reading, and study standing. If you are a tactile learner, the point is not that you must "act out" what
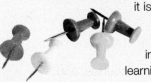
it is you are trying to learn, but that doing any activity or moving while you are learning will help it sink in.

2. Consider your strengths as a student. Do essay tests make you break out in a cold sweat? Are you cool as a cucumber when faced with an oral exam or speaking in front of a group of people? Keep in mind that course content and grade calculation can vary from one course section to another. For instance, if you don't test well, try to locate course options that place more emphasis on papers, projects, or lab assignments versus performance on exams and quizzes. Look carefully at each syllabus you receive or online, in advance if possible, and consider due dates and exams for all your courses. Will they be complementing or competing with each other?

3. Know how you learn. Knowing your learning style can help you make the most of your classes and study time. This is a surefire way to help you do your absolute best and reduce stress and anxiety about underperforming. By this point in your education, you probably have a sense about which style suits you best.

Know Your Options

Consider your current course load and your overall schedule. Is your total number of credits in line with your other time demands? If you are juggling athletics or working long hours, think about the following:

- Cutting back on your course load if it doesn't interfere with graduation requirements
- Cutting back on sports, work, or other extracurricular activities

Look at what you can let go. It may take a semester longer to finish or mean you have to pay back a loan, depending on which choices are best for you. However, this does not mean you are an unsuccessful student, but a responsible one who is realistic about what can be done and done well. Other actions you can take to cope with the stressors of rising to academic expectations include the following:

- Talk to your advisor about how to balance your courses. You might be able to take some electives along with your difficult courses, balancing things out a bit.

- Find a tutor. Your campus probably has a writing center, math lab, and myriad of other resources to help you do your best in courses you are concerned about. Even if you never need to use one of these resources, just knowing they are available to you will ease your mind.

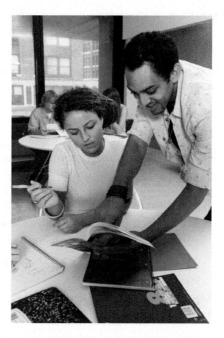

Table 4.1 The ABC's of Getting the Most out of Your Tutor

If you ask a classmate or enlist the help of a tutor, you want to prepare in order to get the most out of the session.

Before:	Write down as many questions you can think of. Evaluate your own strengths and areas where you need to improve and share these with your tutor. Complete assigned work to the best of your ability.
During:	Use text, notes, and class assignments. Write new notes when appropriate. Write down questions to ask instructor. If you need to, ask the tutor to slow down or to repeat a confusing concept.
After:	Review what you learned in your tutoring session. Follow up with your instructor. Plan ahead for your next class and tutor session.

Study Smart

Have you ever sat down to complete a reading assignment, and ten pages into it, you have no idea what you just read? Maybe you have experienced studying for an exam, but no matter what you do the information just won't sink in. Studying in your new and unstructured college environment can be a challenge. You might find yourself stressing because no matter how much time you spend studying, you just can't make the grade.

Your Study Environment

First, it is important to make sure you are studying in an environment that will encourage success. Follow these tips:

- **Location, location, location.** Find a spot that is quiet, just comfortable enough (you don't want study time to turn into nap time), well lit, and absent from such distractions as friends that want to chat, ringing phones, and blaring music. Make this spot your study spot—one you can return to time and time again.

- **Plan your time.** You'll probably find that not all of your classes require the same amount of study time. For example, if you're good at languages, then Spanish class probably doesn't require hours and hours of your concentration. However, if chemistry is giving you a hard time, plan in advance to spend more time with this subject. Allocate more time to difficult classes.

- **Take breaks.** Most of us have an attention span of only so much time, and it is probably less than 30 minutes. Take study breaks and let your mind wander for a few minutes, step outside, or work on something else. Tasks are usually more manageable if we break them up into small chunks, rather than tackling the whole thing all at once. Be logical in how you break up your study sessions. Try to break when you've completed a section or topic. Whatever you do, don't cram.

Study Strategies

Once you've nailed down the perfect study spot, you're ready to develop a strategy. Everyone is different, so what works for you might not work for your best friend. If you're not sure about an effective method for getting the most out of your course materials, start with the SQ4R study method, or **S**urvey, **Q**uestion, **R**ead, **R**ecite, **R**eview, **R**eflect. Once you've learned to use this method, you can tailor it to suit your learning style.

1. **Survey.** This is the first step of SQ4R and gives a sneak preview of the chapter or unit materials. Your goal in this step is to get a general sense of the material you are about to study. If you are studying from a textbook, look at the chapter's headings, and read the objectives and summaries. This information will clue you in to important points when you actually read the material.

2. **Question.** Now that you know what to expect, flip through the chapter again and turn each main heading into a question. For example, if the heading says, "Causes of Alcohol Abuse and Alcoholism," ask yourself, "What are the Causes of Alcohol Abuse and Alcoholism?" This step will make important points stand out, and will further increase your understanding of the material. Record your questions on a sheet of paper.

3. **Read.** The first of the "R's" in "4R." In this step, find answers to the questions you created in step 2. Now you are diving into the actual content, and searching for the answer to a specific question will help you maintain your concentration. Actively searching for a specific answer is much more beneficial than simply reading a section with no specific goal in mind.

4. **Recite.** Now that you've found the answer, write it down in your own words. It is important for you to do this step from memory, so close your book or notebook. If you are having trouble, go back and review the tricky material in your book or notes. Still stuck? Move on and come back to this section later, try rephrasing your original question, or contact your professor to schedule time for extra help.

5. **Review.** Once you've made it through the entire chapter or assignment, review your notes. Check your memory and understanding of the material by reciting answers to your questions or the main points for each heading. A methodical review can include not only this assignment, but older assignments too, especially if you have a big exam coming up. Reviewing what you know in your own words is a very effective method for retaining information and helping you get the main points of the assignment.

6. **Reflect.** What types of conclusions can you draw from this chapter? Do you have new questions or ideas about this material? Compare your own ideas to the ones from the assignment, and note any answers to additional questions you have, or differences between your ideas. How do your ideas or questions fall into the organization of the chapter or assignment? Record this organization, and relate the main concepts to your pre-existing knowledge or to examples from your own life.

Test Success

It's no secret that tests can be one of the most stressful parts of being a college student. For some classes, how you perform on an exam could make up the majority of your grade. For some students, doing well on an exam is their chance to let the instructor know they take the class seriously and understand the material. You can be proactive in preparing yourself for test day, beyond reviewing the material you learned in class.

Ask your professor questions about the exam

Your instructor wants you to succeed. Don't be afraid to spend some time going over the following questions with your instructor as you develop a study plan:

- How many items or questions will there be?
- What types of questions can I expect? (multiple choice, true/false, essay)
- What material does the exam cover?
- How much does the exam count toward my grade?
- Is there a time limit?

Ask yourself questions as you prepare for the exam

- What other obligations do I have the week of the exam?
- How much time will I need to spend studying and reviewing?
- How will this change my current schedule?

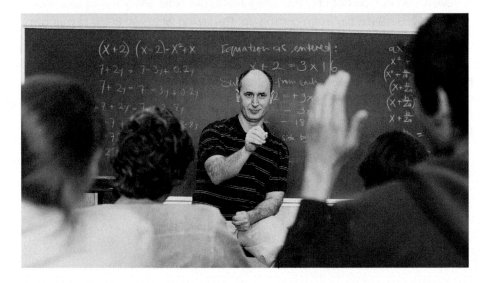

Reduce Exam Stress

Reviewing and preparing for a test involves more than reading over your notes. Plan ahead for study time by setting aside at least an hour everyday for a study session. Develop a strategy that boosts your confidence and assures you that you know the material. Ask a roommate to quiz you, take advantage of practice test questions that are at the end of your book's chapter or provided by the professor, or draw pictures and create lyrics or mnemonic devices that help you remember information. Creating summaries and making use of flash cards are also excellent methods of preparing for test day.

Coping with test stress

Sometimes, no matter how well prepared you might be, test anxiety can catch up with you. Use the following strategies to improve your game plan on test day.

1. **Visualize all possible outcomes.** This way, you will feel prepared and not surprised. Anticipate any potential problems and how to handle them effectively. If your roommate isn't available and you need someone to quiz you, have a backup plan. Imagine getting to the exam early to sit where you will be least distracted by latecomers or those who finish early. Go in knowing your strengths and weaknesses.

2. **Talk to yourself.** If you think, "I am not ready for this test—I shouldn't be taking it," catch yourself and say, "I am well prepared and I am ready to do my best."

3. **Have a plan.** On exam day or the day of a presentation, have a routine. Eat a good breakfast; exercise; review a small part of the material, but not too much; and focus on things to relax you. Review how you'll arrive early and where you'll sit, and take a few deep breaths. Start your routine the night before with plenty of rest and good nutrition.

4. **Plan an attack.** Find out the number of and types of questions before the test if possible. Calculate how much time each question should take you, but don't watch the clock. Read through all the questions when you get the test. If you get stuck on a question, don't spend extra time on it; circle it so you can come back at the end if need be. Do answer those challenging questions you want to come back to, rather than leave them blank.

5. **Finish strong.** Don't think you're doing poorly if people finish before you. Calmly remind yourself that you are taking your time. Anticipate this happening, and sit where you'll be less distracted if it does. Check that all questions are completed and your name or identification number is on the exam before you hand it in.

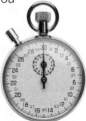

Table 4.2 Signs Of Test Day Stress

Mental	Physical
Decreased attention span	Shortness of breath
Confusion	Muscle tension
Forgetfulness	Elevated pulse or blood pressure
Rapid speech	Nausea, upset stomach
Irritability	Diarrhea, need to urinate

Presentations

Take the symptoms of test day stress times five, and you have the classic symptoms of stage fright! Touted as the number one fear of the majority of all people, it can paralyze you before a speech or presentation, but only if you let it!

If you've stood at the front of a room with dry mouth, sweaty hands, fast pulse, shaky knees, and trembling legs, you know stage fright firsthand. Breaking down stage fright is a first step in reducing it. Completely eliminating it probably isn't realistic and, surprisingly, is not necessarily your goal. Fear actually sharpens your reflexes, heightens your energy, and adds a spark to your presentations.

Combat your fear and become an expert presenter

- Several days before the presentation, you may not feel very nervous and may lack a sense of urgency to prepare for your presentation.

  Solutions: Prepare, have a passion for what you are talking about, rehearse in front of someone or videotape yourself, organize your notes, and absolutely memorize your opening statement so you start strong and feel good about it.

- Right before the speech, you will probably be the most nervous. Focus on ways to keep calm.

  Solutions: Don't rush; allow yourself ample time to get there so you don't add the anxiety of being late to the mix. This will also give you a chance to survey your surrounding and get comfortable with the setup. Finally, greet your audience as they enter, converse with one or two of them, and breathe deep.

- During the speech, you'll probably start to relax a bit and find that you are feeling much better.

  Solutions: Find friendly faces in the audience to focus on, joke about your nerves, let the audience see that you're human, and plant notes around the stage or podium so you will have reminders if you get stuck.

The top five presentation don'ts to avoid

1. **Don't say "sorry."** If you misspeak, or stumble as you are getting started, don't apologize. Just take it in stride and move on.

2. **Stay Focused.** Don't stare down at the ground, your feet, your hands, the podium, or the like. Pick a friendly face, or a spot on the wall at the back of the room, and stick with it. If you can manage, survey the room as you speak and try to make eye contact with various individuals.

3. **Don't say "um."**

4. **Make eye contact with your audience.** Avoid reading directly from your notes.

5. **Watch your tone.** Try to speak as though you were actually talking with someone, and avoid getting stuck in a monotone speech pattern. A conversational tone will spice things up and engage your audience.

Group presentations

Working in a group to prepare and present information can be both rewarding and frustrating. The benefits of sharing ideas and sharing the workload can be diminished when a group member fails to carry his or her load. Thorough planning, adequate prep time, and open communication among all group members are keys for a successful group experience. It is a good idea to create an outline of duties and responsibilities complete with a timeline that each group member agrees on.

- As a group, list what needs to be done and the order in which tasks need to be completed.

- Divide the workload into equal shares based on the number in your group, and assign each group member a role.

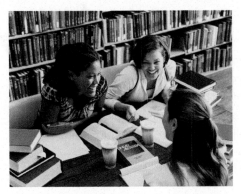

Staying on task and communicating with your team members is key to a successful group project.

- Determine how and when you will share information. Will you e-mail, meet in person, or both?

- Lastly, how and when will you practice the presentation of the information? You may be graded individually or as a group, but keep in mind that your collaborative use of the information is key to a successful group presentation.

48

Beating Stress with Exercise

Your pulse is racing, you're breathing faster, and you're sweating right through your shirt. Are you working out or stressing out? Your body's response to stress can be very similar to its response to strenuous exercise. Exercise can become an effective stress reducer for you, in part for that very reason. Ever notice that you aren't nearly as bothered by your roommate's loud voice or clothes on the floor if you've had a good workout? But if you haven't made time for exercise lately, even the slightest annoyance can agitate you. Here's why:

- Exercise encourages the brain's production of "feel-good" hormones that calm you back down to handle stress more effectively. Whether you're on the elliptical, the basketball court, or the floor of a yoga class, your body is fighting stress in ways science is just beginning to understand.

- Exercise helps your body respond better to stressful situations. Because the body's responses to exercise and stress are so similar, experts believe that your body is much better prepared to face life beyond the gym if you are active.

- Exercise and physical activity provides opportunities for social support. Recreational activities (kickball, ultimate frisbee, jogging with a friend) encourage a sense of fun and play with other individuals that have similar interests and can provide a number opportunities to discuss the low points of your day, along with the high points. The sharing that ensues, ensures one that they are not alone and that help is available for the asking.

- Exercise is like moving meditation. Certain forms of exercise (cross-country skiing, swimming, hiking, bicycling) require a fairly consistent repetitive motion, which can alter your state of mind. Experts call it moving meditation, and the physiological effects of regular participation in these activities are very similar to what happens when one practices meditation. The repetitive acts of breathing and movement associated with certain activities act as a mantra, and may in part be responsible for the feelings of calmness and tranquility following a satisfying exercise session.

- Exercise can alleviate muscular tension. During stress, muscles contract and loose their normal resting muscle tone. Physical activity puts tense muscles to work, and releases that pent-up energy and allows muscle groups to return to their normal state. Physical activity might just relieve that pain in your neck caused by hunching over your books for too many hours, or a tension headache brought on by the argument you had with your roommate last night.

Exactly how exercise affects your personal stress level depends on several factors. Your physical status, the intensity of the exercise, and your feelings about exercise all play a role. Most importantly, choose an activity you enjoy. Your activity of choice should be time to forget the day's worries and just focus on you.

Choosing a Type of Exercise

Deciding which type of stress-busting activity is best for you can be mind-boggling. The good news: any form of exercise can give you a psychological lift that beats stress. It all boils down to what you enjoy. So, don't add to your stress by agonizing over which activity to choose. If you are also looking for a way to improve your overall level of fitness, aerobic exercise might be a good choice for you. If you want to flash toned muscles along with your stress-free attitude, resistance training is a good option. Mind-body activities such as yoga and tai chi are often associated with stress reduction, and are more obvious options, but the choice is yours.

The No-Stress Approach to Incorporating Activity into Your Life

Already time crunched and worried that fitting exercise into your life will add more stress? Start slowly, and don't worry about missing out on a day or two. Take a "life's messy" approach. Give yourself space to be busy with other aspects of your life at times without feeling like you've fallen off the wagon. There is no need for mega-activity in order to reduce stress.

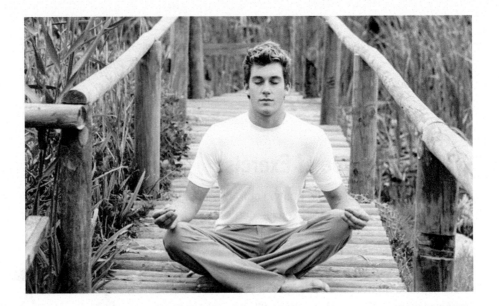

Incorporate mind-body exercise

Mind-body exercise includes yoga, tai chi, and other Eastern-origin exercise. How can you incorporate these styles of activity into your life?

- Search for a local yoga studio or a community center that offers classes, or check out your school's physical education offerings.
- Consider a dance class. Like Eastern-based exercise, dance can be a fun way to forget your worries.
- Try meditation. Pick a quiet spot that gives you good vibes, take some deep breaths, and clear your mind. Though you aren't exercising here, you are performing an activity that will help you relax and can improve the rest of your day.
- Try the relaxation exercises at the end of this chapter.

Mind-body modes of exercise have been linked to better memory, mood, sleep quality, concentration, and to increased energy levels—all crucial to your success as a student, and all compromised if you are under stress.

How to Stress-Proof Yourself through Exercise

- Even 10 minutes at a moderate pace can boost your mood. As you improve, or are less busy, aim for 30 to 60 minutes at least 5 days a week. To avoid injury, increase slowly, adding 2 minutes a week to your time.
- Choose something you enjoy so your exercise routine isn't something you dread and backfires by adding stress to your life.

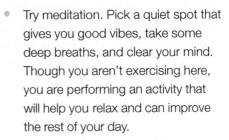

Traditional forms of exercise

It might not surprise you that running, weight lifting, or playing basketball can also produce mind-body experiences. A runner who enjoys the breeze on her skin and the rhythm of her feet hitting the ground without worrying about how far or how fast knows there's no need for a yoga mat to decompress.

A Get-Started Guide for Any Personality Type

Are you competitive?

Choose from a variety of team or individual sports such as basketball, racquetball, or intramural football. Enter road races or contests. Set time or distance goals for yourself to provide a competitive edge that you will enjoy.

Are you less competitive?

Perform activities where you can get lost in the process. Walk or bike outdoors on your own, but in a safe place. Or you might prefer to use the cardio equipment at the gym, where you can go at your own pace.

Are you social?

Choose group activities that might also include laid-back team sports like ultimate frisbee, or kickball, or choose dance or group fitness classes. You can find clubs for various interests from martial arts to triathlon training that will provide you with workout partners as well as a support group.

Are you more introverted?

Use your time on the elliptical to read a magazine or plug into your iPod. Lift weights and focus on your inner strength at the same time. Try a variety of aerobic, yoga, or Pilates videos on your own. Peaceful walks outside would also be a stress-free exercise option for you.

Are you aggressive?

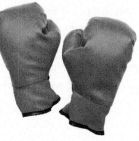

Try aerobic kickboxing or boxing. Lift weights with a workout partner who will encourage and push you. You might also enjoy the same types of activities as those who are competitive, so team sports like football and basketball might be right up your alley.

Don't make exercise a source of stress

No matter what your personality type is, remember that whichever activity you choose should be something you can enjoy. If you're starting out on a routine to reduce stress, try and keep the activity in perspective and focus on the moment. Focusing on a game of basketball, or keeping up with your group fitness instructor's steps, draws your attention from life's problems and clears your mind. The simple act of distracting yourself from the routine of your day can help you feel better later, so avoid worrying about physical results while you're working out. If you do choose physical activity with a specific weight or fitness goal in mind, your routine could become counter productive. Be sure to have a carefully balanced approach to physical activity if you use exercise to achieve a fitness goal and as a source of stress relief.

Sun Salutations

You don't have to break a sweat to reap the benefits of some physical activity. Try these quick exercises first thing in the morning to start your day off right.

- Stretch in the shower. The hot water will loosen up your muscles, making it easier to get a good stretch. Not only will a nice, deep stretch feel great, but it will help you release stored tension and enable you to start the day feeling more relaxed, at peace, and ready to handle what comes your way.

- Go for a morning walk. Whether it is around the block, or a brisk-paced 1 mile walk, the health benefits abound, making the stress management benefits the cherry on top! A morning walk can get you ready for your day, help you sleep better at night, lower your stress level, and reduce your risk of numerous health conditions. A morning walk will get your blood pumping, and give you a chance to clear your mind for the day ahead. Give it a try!

- Do some yoga. You don't have to be a yoga expert to experience the healthy body and peaceful mind yoga encourages. Combining all the benefits of several stress management techniques, such as diaphragmic breathing, meditation, stretching, and more, yoga provides some of the best stress management and health benefits you can find in a single technique. A good way to start your morning is by doing a series of yoga poses called Sun Salutations. Not sure where to find information to help you get started on your new morning yoga ritual? Check out www.abc-of-yoga.com.

Relaxation Exercises

For one reason or another, we might not always have the time to go for a half-hour walk, a quick run, or hit the gym. A brief session of progressive muscle relaxation or visual imagery can help us relax and get some of the same stress-busting benefits as actual exercise. If you have a few minutes of time and are in need of a stress reducing "quickie," help is here.

Progressive muscle relaxation

You can practice progressive relaxation exercises in isolation (one body part only) or from toe to head. When you feel tension in your neck and shoulders, for instance, but can't take the time to lie down and truly relax completely, just follow the steps for shoulders and neck. If you can't sleep, get comfortable and perform the entire exercise from start to finish.

1. Inhale and tighten your toes; Exhale and relax your toes.
2. Inhale and tighten your feet; Exhale and relax your feet.
3. Inhale and tighten your ankles; Exhale and relax your ankles.
4. Inhale and tighten your hamstrings and quadriceps; Exhale and relax your hamstrings and quadriceps.
5. Inhale and tighten your gluteals (buttocks); Exhale and relax your gluteals.
6. Inhale and tighten your abdominals; Exhale and relax your abdominals.
7. Inhale and expand through your chest; Exhale and relax your chest.
8. Inhale and raise your shoulders up to your neck; Exhale and relax your shoulders and neck.
9. Inhale and make fists with your hands; Exhale and relax your hands.
10. Inhale and tighten your arm; Exhale and relax your arms.
11. Inhale and smile as wide as you can; Exhale and let your face relax.
12. Inhale and raise your eyebrows as high as you can; Exhale and allow your eyebrows to return to their resting place.
13. Inhale and mentally scan your body for any sources of remaining tension; Exhale and allow that tension to drain from your body.

Guided imagery skills to relieve stress

Visualizing images that you associate with comfort reduces stress levels. Read through the following guided imagery exercise, and then close your eyes and review the exercise. You might also try recording your voice so that you can play it back. Transform yourself with your own imagery to a place that is relaxing and rejuvenating for you. Try to use as many senses as you can. Find a comfortable position and begin.

Breathe in and out slowly, evenly, and deeply.

Imagine yourself . . . in a meadow . . . at the mountains . . . on the beach . . .

Imagine the luscious surroundings . . . the brilliant sky and the deep shades of the trees . . . the deep turquoise of the water against the sand . . .

Feel the warmth of the sun on your skin . . . just warm enough to feel good . . .

Breathe in and out.

Feel a gentle breeze around you, lightly touching your arms and face . . .

Hear the sounds of the surroundings . . . the birds . . . leaves gently blowing in the trees . . . water running down a stream . . . ocean waves coming in and retreating . . .

Breathe in and out. Enjoy the warmth of the sun.

Take in the smells around you . . . the grasses and fresh new flowers . . . the crisp clean air and evergreens . . . the salty ocean spray . . .

Breathe in and out with the sun warming you, and the breeze alternately keeping you cool and comfortable.

Breathe in completely and then exhale fully and completely. Allow yourself to be completely absorbed in the place you're seeing.

Relationships

Combating
Conflict and the
Stress that Comes with It

It's 2 A.M. and, you are sound asleep in bed. Your roommate bursts through the door with two other people, and they proceed to gossip and munch on potato chips, while you toss and turn in hopes they'll notice you and leave. Sound familiar?

On a daily basis you interact with roommates, classmates, professors, coworkers, significant others, friends, and family. All of these interactions aren't bound to be positive, and the negative exchanges can be a significant source of stress. So how can you address your roommate when she barges through the door in the middle of the night with others in tow all the time? What's the best way to approach your significant other to have an "I think we should see other people" talk? This chapter will take you through some steps that will help you dance with ease through relationship conflict and keep your stress level under control.

Dealing with Personality Differences

Do you suffer from "samesightedness"? Have you ever had a disagreement with someone to no avail, because each of you has a completely different point of view? Recognizing who you are and acknowledging that others might just have a different opinion because of fundamental differences in culture, beliefs, or values are steps in minimizing stressful relationship conflict. Remember these three things:

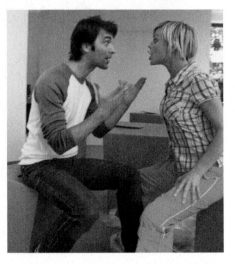

- Most people aren't going to be, think, or act just like you!
- Acknowledge personality differences in others to become more effective in your communication. You might think things over, while your roommate might make spontaneous decisions.
- Good friends and people you get along with easily probably have a very similar personality to yours. You'll have to work harder to get along with those who are less like you.

Top Ten Communication Offenses

Can you survive the relationship police? No matter what your personality, in order to relate to someone, you have to be interested more than interesting. Are you guilty of these Top 10 Communication Offenses? If you are, then use the *Get out of Jail* suggestion that follows each offense to help you improve your connections with people today!

1. **Talking more than listening.**

   Get out of jail: Listen more than you talk. Ask questions instead of jumping in with advice or solutions.

2. **Interrupting when someone else is talking.**

   Get out of jail: Let them finish. Cutting someone off indicates you don't really care about the message. Waiting to speak up signals that you are listening and thoughtful of the other person's feelings or opinion.

3. **Looking anywhere but at the person talking.**

   Get out of jail: Make eye contact, and turn to face the speaker.

Relationship Conflict Survival Tips

Let's say you are having a conflict with your roommate. What do you do so that you can focus on upcoming exams and study without the added stress of tiptoeing around or avoiding them? There are some steps to take that will make it bearable and might flex your relationship-building muscles at the same time.

- Recognize that challenges happen in all relationships.

- Identify the source of stress. Take time to narrow it down to one specific thing.

- Make a plan that includes awareness of your own verbal and nonverbal reactions that make matters worse. No yelling, shutting down, or becoming too emotional; uncross your arms, don't slam doors, take those hands off your hips, and no heavy sighs.

- Calm down by taking a deep breath, counting to ten, or literally waiting a day or two if you need to cool down before addressing the conflict.

- Tackle one issue at a time. Trying to fix everything at once creates more problems. Instead of "Can you not trash the place all the time," try "Will you please clean up the kitchen and wipe off the counter when you are done?"

- Avoid personal attacks. "You're a messy slob" is judgmental. Target a problematic behavior or action. "Last night the dishes were a mile high."

- Acknowledge improvements or even effort made in the right direction. "The kitchen looks great this week; I really appreciate it."

- Follow through with shared positive experiences. Make an effort to share a meal, go to a ballgame or concert, or plan study breaks together during finals week.

When to Talk and When to Listen

Try the following acronyms to buff up your relationships.

W.A.I.T. stands for "Why am I talking?" Know how you are going to contribute to the conversation before you open your mouth. Consider what you are going to say and how it affects someone else.

C.A.R.E.

Concentrate on what is being said as well as what is not being said, the nonverbal messages. Fast or slower rate of speech? Eye contact? Long pauses? Body language?

Acknowledge that you are listening. Nod and send other encouragers.

Restate what's said in your own words to confirm that the person is being heard. "If I hear you correctly, what you are saying is . . ."

Empathize by revealing sensitivity to feelings. "I can understand how that would make you frustrated."

4. **Fidgeting or multitasking while someone is talking.**

   Get out of jail: Be still and focus. Fidgety behavior might convey the message that you just can't wait for the conversation to be over!

5. **Making no facial expressions.**

   Get out of jail: Respond with a smile, a look of concern, or a raised eyebrow.

6. **Never smiling.**

   Get out of jail: Smile more. No one likes a sour-puss!

7. **Asking questions about what was just said that prove you aren't listening.**

   Get out of jail: Ask questions to clarify, but listen well enough not to need a repeat.

8. **Turning whatever someone else says into something all about you.**

   Get out of jail: Avoid using *I* when you respond. Although "I understand" is helpful, too often "I" statements launch into self-centered stories. Focus on listening instead of speaking.

9. **Finishing someone's sentences.**

   Get out of jail: Don't assume you know what someone is going to say. As with interrupting, a person could interpret that you don't really care to hear his or her complete thought.

10. **Looking at your watch while someone is talking.**

    Get out of jail: Resist, or stop them and let them know how little time you have and how important this is to you. Then reschedule when you have more time to listen.

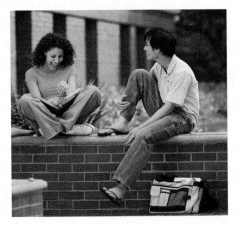

Romance: Coping with the Stress and Challenges That Come with It

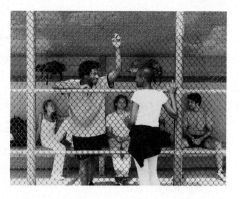

Susan's boyfriend, John, was overwhelmed from writing term papers, studying for exams, and sending out applications for summer work. She had been used to more frequent attention and missed talking to him. When he finally called her, she was angry instead of letting him know she was glad to hear from him. He was surprised and disappointed in her reaction, and bothered that she lacked understanding. Once the stress of being overly busy and being separated ends, the stress of miscommunication lingers! How could they have avoided this?

The communication gap

- Susan wanted more assurance from John while he was busy.
- Susan was projecting that John was disinterested in her because he was distracted by other things that were taking his time.
- John expected Susan to know how stressed and focused he was on all he had to do.
- John wanted to stay on task and get done in order to see Susan when he was finished.

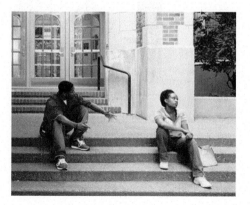

The fix

- Let your partner know what you need to do. John could have asked for time and space to get his work done.
- Ask your partner what you can do to help. Susan would have learned that by not being needy or unhappy, she would be helping John have more energy to get things done.

You and your parents are arguing over whether or not you should go to Cancún for spring break. How do you talk it out without turning it into a huge argument and a source of stress?

Talking is the easy part. If you consider a few details, you'll get better results.

- What do you actually want from the message you're going to send? You want to go to Mexico. You want your parents to give their consent, if not their financial help! You want them to listen to you without saying "no" to the idea before hearing you out.

- Who are you talking to, and how do they process information? Your parents are likely to be concerned about your safety and the details of your trip and traveling companions. The financial details will be important to them. Present your solution to cost objections before they come up.

What could get in your way? If you already anticipate resistance and begin with an emotional plea, you'll only get what you most fear! Do your homework. How much are the tickets? Where will you stay? Who will be with you? Make your case: explain your position, and accept that there will be questions. Field them by responding, not reacting defensively. If all goes well, you can pack your bags and send a postcard!

62

- Go by the facts, and don't let your insecurities run wild. Susan felt ignored even when she knew what was taking John's time. She was projecting insecurities into the situation that weren't justified.

- Find other interests outside of your relationships. Susan could have taken the time to pursue other activities, call her friends, catch up on movies or her own homework, or exercise.

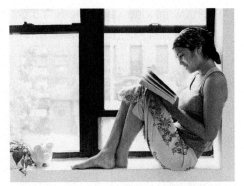

Independence and the ability to enjoy alone-time is important for any healthy relationship.

Classroom Conflict

You have to take a course that is a prerequisite for your major. You've already heard that the professor is condescending and unapproachable. The class is a large lecture, and the grade is based on two exams. After just a few classes, you are worried that you are not going to do well. How do you forge a relationship with this hands-off professor and get the most out of this class?

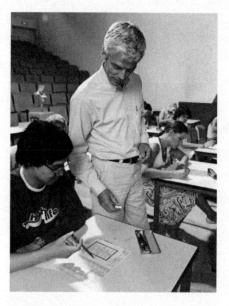

- Explore your options. Believing that alternatives exist is critical. This may be the only class section you can take, but developing a way to relate to the professor, or how you cope with the stress of the situation, can help. Feeling trapped and without choice is the greatest stressor of all.

- Understand that the professor may not realize that his failure to provide any direction or feedback makes him a bad teacher for some students. He may think he is empowering you to explore concepts on your own, or he may be so overwhelmed by the numbers of students in large lectures that he can't provide support for each individually.

- Talk to this professor, and discuss your concerns and options. Be polite and focus on your needs. Relay that you want to have a thorough understanding of the material, not just get a passing grade. Ask for his recommendations for additional practice, a tutor, or volunteer work that will reinforce the course work.

- If all else fails, go to your advisor for help. Document the steps you have already taken to make improvements. This step may change the relationship you have with a professor entirely, so be sure you have explored all other options first.

Stress-Busting Products and Services

A Closer Look

Stress—we've all got it, and products and services that promise to reduce or eliminate your stress are a multimillion-dollar industry. So, how do you know what really works, and what might be a waste of your money? In college, stress is a common part of life, and sometimes you might need just a little extra help coping with all the challenges that come your way. In this chapter, we'll look at some popular alternative stress-busting approaches that might just work, and how you can apply them to your everyday life. We'll also take a look at the gimmicks you might come across on late-night television infomercials, and the questions you should ask yourself before dialing that 1-800 number.

Looking at Products That Promise to Relieve Your Stress

If a claim sounds too good to be true, it probably is! Consider the following before you buy:

1. Use discretion when selecting alternative therapies or natural remedies that are not yet regulated by government agencies. Because a growing number of new ideas are still being researched, it can be difficult to sort through what is actually research based and what is being marketed by someone wanting to make a quick buck.

2. Be wary of products that proclaim they are "innovative," a "quick cure," or an "exclusive product." Something that is truly a breakthrough cure for disease would be widely reported. That said, the words *suppressed by the Government* is most likely a gimmick used by advertisers to make their product appear to be a best-kept secret.

3. Be aware of any false beliefs you may have. Myths about herbal remedies are plentiful. "If a product won't help, it won't hurt." All chemicals can be toxic. Don't believe that "natural means healthy and safe." Being natural or herbal doesn't make something safe. Not well-defined or controlled, these terms on a label are used to imply unsubstantiated benefits or safety. The bottom line is that though many herbal or natural remedies have potential, the evidence is often inconclusive.

Natural (and Free!) Strategies for Busting Stress

Healthy pleasures like beautiful sights, fragrance, and music are all recognized for their ability to reduce stress and to enhance well-being. You can safely put them and a few others to work for you!

Table 7.1 Color Connections

Use this color . . .	To achieve this effect . . .
Red	Associated with energy, increased pulse, and increased stimulation. Wear it to the gym.
Green	The most relaxing color for your brain. It heals and soothes, but also helps focus. Include green in the color scheme of the room where you study; buy green notebooks; wear green to your next exam.
Blue	Another calming color. If you are anxious before an exam or presentation, look at the sky, a body of water, or even close your eyes and simply visualize it.
Violet	A calming color that can help create deep relaxation. Buy sheets, comforters, or pajamas, or add a poster in your bedroom, featuring violet.

Color therapy

When should you wear red? Why do talk show guests wait in the "green room"? How can the color of your folders be important? Color has the power to stir emotions and affects the brain faster than speech or the written word, that's how. Every color affects emotion differently because of how they affect different parts of your brain. Bright, intense hues stimulate the limbic system in the brain, which controls emotion.

Aromatherapy

Your sense of smell is your most primal sense because aromas go straight to your brain and smell is registered with every breath you take. Your limbic system (or "emotion central") is stimulated by smell, and will trigger your reactions and instincts. Lemon and lavender are two of the safest essential oils to begin experimenting with. To safely put aromatherapy to work for you,

- be sure you are using 100% pure essential oils.

- only use it in the dilution concentration suggested on the bottle. Health food markets can help if you have questions.

- understand the difference between pure essential oils and other products that you might buy. Synthetics in many products can cause allergic reactions or sensitivity.

"Scentsational" Strategies

- To relax before bed, mix three to nine drops of lavender essential oil with sea salt or honey. Add to a tubful of water by swirling under running water. Relax in the bath, or simply enjoy the aroma.

- Instead of caffeine as a pick-me-up in the afternoon, try drinking lemon water. Just squeeze some fresh lemon in your water to refresh, energize, and enhance digestion.

- To enhance your mental acuity, try an aromatherapy diffuser using lemon essential oil. Diffusers vaporize and disperse essential oils directly into the air. They are an investment, though, so you might want to try one out before buying. Alternatively, you can try scented candles to achieve the same effect.

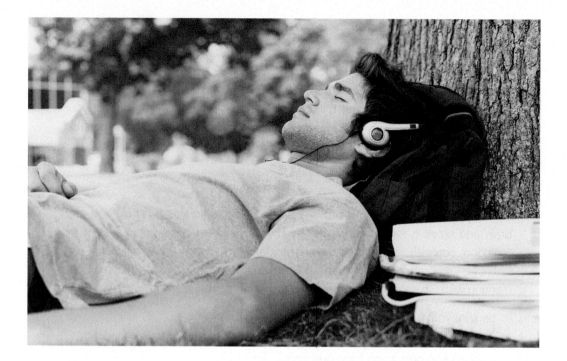

Music therapy

The soothing ability of music can be a powerful stress buster. Select music and sounds can enhance your studying, workouts, and daily routine. Calm down, rev up, and refresh your nervous system all through your choice of music. Music is so motivationally powerful, in fact, that the use of iPods has been ruled illegal in some competitive races. Some race commissioners believe that the athlete with an iPod has an unfair advantage.

Experiment with music and your mood. When you feel anxious, play classical or more sedative music with a slow tempo. Keep the volume low to calm and refresh your nerves if you are tense. Beethoven's *Symphony No. 6*, a tape recording of sea sounds, or music intended for yoga or meditation would all be good sounds to soothe.

To increase heart rate and prepare for physical activity, you may often intuitively do the opposite by playing faster, louder music.

Breathing

All you really have to do today is breathe in, breathe out. When you have nothing else, you still have a powerful tool. Yoga is 7,000 years old, and it is still going strong. While you can't go into down dog in your lecture hall, you can use many breathing techniques employed in yoga to affect your state of mind.

Before an exam . . .

Inhale and exhale through your left nostril by closing your right gently. Repeat ten times for relaxation. When you repeat the above on your right nostril, you'll be tapping into your analytical side, and better able to concentrate and focus on fact.

To relieve a headache . . .

Inhale through your left nostril, then exhale through the right. Repeat five times. Inhale through the right nostril, then exhale through the left. Repeat five times.

When you can't fall asleep because your mind is racing . . .

Breathe naturally. Make no effort to control it. Simply focus on how your body responds to each inhale and exhale. Practice mindful and effortless breathing. Repeat ten times.

What Is Meditation?

Though you probably have heard of it, do you know how to do it? The practice of meditation is about shifting focus from your busy outer world of classes, exams, and social functions, and directing it inward. The challenge for you in meditation is to quiet your incessantly "chattering mind." Instead of thinking of the past or the future, what has or what will happen, meditation promotes being in the present moment. It can last for 20 minutes, as some experts recommend, or 2, but will reap you more benefits as you make it a daily practice. Three focusing techniques here introduce you to meditation.

Before you begin

- Sit with an erect spine. Sit in a chair, or cross-legged on the floor.
- Find a quiet environment.
- Be open to the experience without needing to control it.

Now you are ready to start

1. **Watch your breath.** Mentally "follow" your breath as it flows in and out of your body. Focus on the space between the inhalation and the exhalation. Your mind may naturally wander; as it does, simply bring it back to the breath.

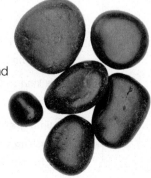

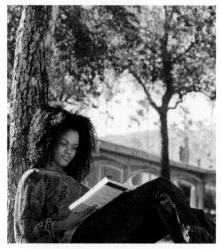

Taking some time out to read a good book or relax in a natural setting is a great stress-buster.

2. Concentrate on an object. Focus on a real object such as a flower, a candle flame, or something in nature. Begin practicing for 5 minutes at a time, concentrating on the object. Extend the time you practice as you become more able to stay completely focused.

3. Recite a mantra. *Mantra* means "control of the mind." To practice mantra meditation, repeat a special word or series of words to help you discipline your mind. You can come up with a string of your own words or use *joy, peace, bliss.*

When should you practice meditation? While you can try it anytime that works for you,

Use Spiritual Rituals to Combat Stress

- Spend time alone every day. Be silent, listen to music, or be in nature.

- Teach someone something; share your talents.

- Keep a journal. Use inspirational quotes, verses, feelings about events and relationships, and ideas. Write about anything that comes to mind, but write fast and be nonjudgmental.

- Volunteer your time for a good cause.

- Read a book that helps you know yourself better or that enriches you.

- Take time out. One day a week, disconnect from technology. Turn off your cell phone, your computer, and your beeper. During this time be alone, or with your family or your friends, but not planning or working on homework. Just be.

- Explore somewhere you have never been before.

- Find joy in small things every day. Watch a baby laugh, or a puppy run; laugh out loud for no reason at all.

- Do a kind act for someone without expecting acknowledgement or anything in return.

- Begin a gratitude list. This could be in conjunction with your journal, or become something that you share with someone else in a letter. Express your appreciation for the gifts in your life: the people, events, and opportunities.

specific times will reap more benefits, say meditation experts. Following vigorous exercise is not an ideal time because it is difficult to abandon the focus on the body. *Before* exercise or following a relaxing yoga session would be better. If you practice before you begin to write a paper or study for an exam, meditation can help clear your mind and create a "zone" of focused awareness around your task.

Stress Busting Gone Bad: Your Questions Answered

What types of herbal remedies can help me reduce stress? Do they work?

Like any medicine, there can be side effects to some alternative therapies. Some herbal remedies, for instance, have proven to be toxic or harmful. St. John's Wort, used as treatment for depression, renders certain drugs ineffective. Kava, used for insomnia, stress, or anxiety, has been linked to liver damage. Simply because something hasn't been found to have known side effects doesn't make it safe until a time when it has been approved by the Food and Drug Association (FDA). Be cautious. Other herbs, or herbal remedies, that claim to reduce stress include feverfew, valerian, and teas with additional ingredients such as skullcap, lemon verbena, and passion flower. While some herbs may be on the FDA's Generally Recognized as Safe (GRAS) list, don't mix herbs with medications. Always check with your physician first.

Why do some people turn to food when they are stressed? What can I do to avoid becoming a stress eater?

Food nurtures, transforms, and comforts. You can have strong emotions tied to food. A preoccupation with food and memories surrounding certain foods can cause problems like binge eating during times of high stress. When was the last time you ate a pint of Chunky Monkey and felt good about it afterward? There is nothing wrong with indulging in a treat, but make sure that you are aware of the choice you are making so you do not feel guilty later. Other things like calling a friend, listening to music, exercising,

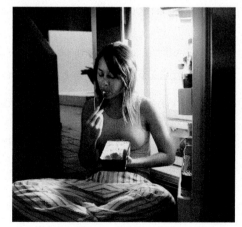

or even yelling might all be things that, at the least, you wouldn't be sorry about after and, at the best, would actually make you feel better right away.

Are there any ways I can use food to control stress that actually may work?

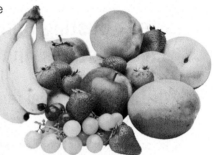

There are many dietary trends emerging. One alternative therapy involves dealing with specific dietary recommendations aimed at finding the right pH balance for your body. The premise is that if your body is not at an optimal pH level, you will struggle more with colds, flu, or allergy symptoms. Because bacteria tend to thrive in acidic environments, researchers say you should eat more high alkaline foods. These include most fresh fruits and vegetables. Foods should be chosen from both sides of the acidic/alkaline food chart, but if you are out of balance, the emphasis should be on alkaline foods.

To enhance your pH balance:

- Add a serving of fruit with each meal. An orange or grapefruit at breakfast, an apple at lunch, and a banana for dinner immediately incorporate alkaline items into your diet.

- You might also want to reduce or limit your intake of alcohol, which is highly acidic.

- Meat, nuts, butter, pasta, beans, coffee, and soda are examples of other acidic foods. You don't have to eliminate them completely; just consider how big a proportion they have in your diet. Then try to balance the scale a little more.

- Artificial sweeteners, as well as sugars, are acidic.

- Antibiotics and other medications are also acidic.

Whether or not this therapy does actually work, tuning into it is in alignment with good nutrition practices, and a strong body does equal a strong mind that is ready to take on life and all the surprises that come with it.

References

American Academy of Family Physicians. 2005. Stress: How to cope better with life's challenges. July. http://familydoctor.org/167.xml.

American Psychological Association. 2004. Exercise fuels the brain's stress buffers. http://www.apa-helpcenter.org/articles/article.php?id=25.

Jim, J. 1990. *Relationship selling: The key to getting and keeping customers.* New York: Penguin.

Robinson, F. P. 1970. *Effective Study,* 4th ed. New York: Harper & Row.

Worksheets on pages 3–5: Courtesy of Karen L. Petersen, Karen@mymorethanmoney.net.